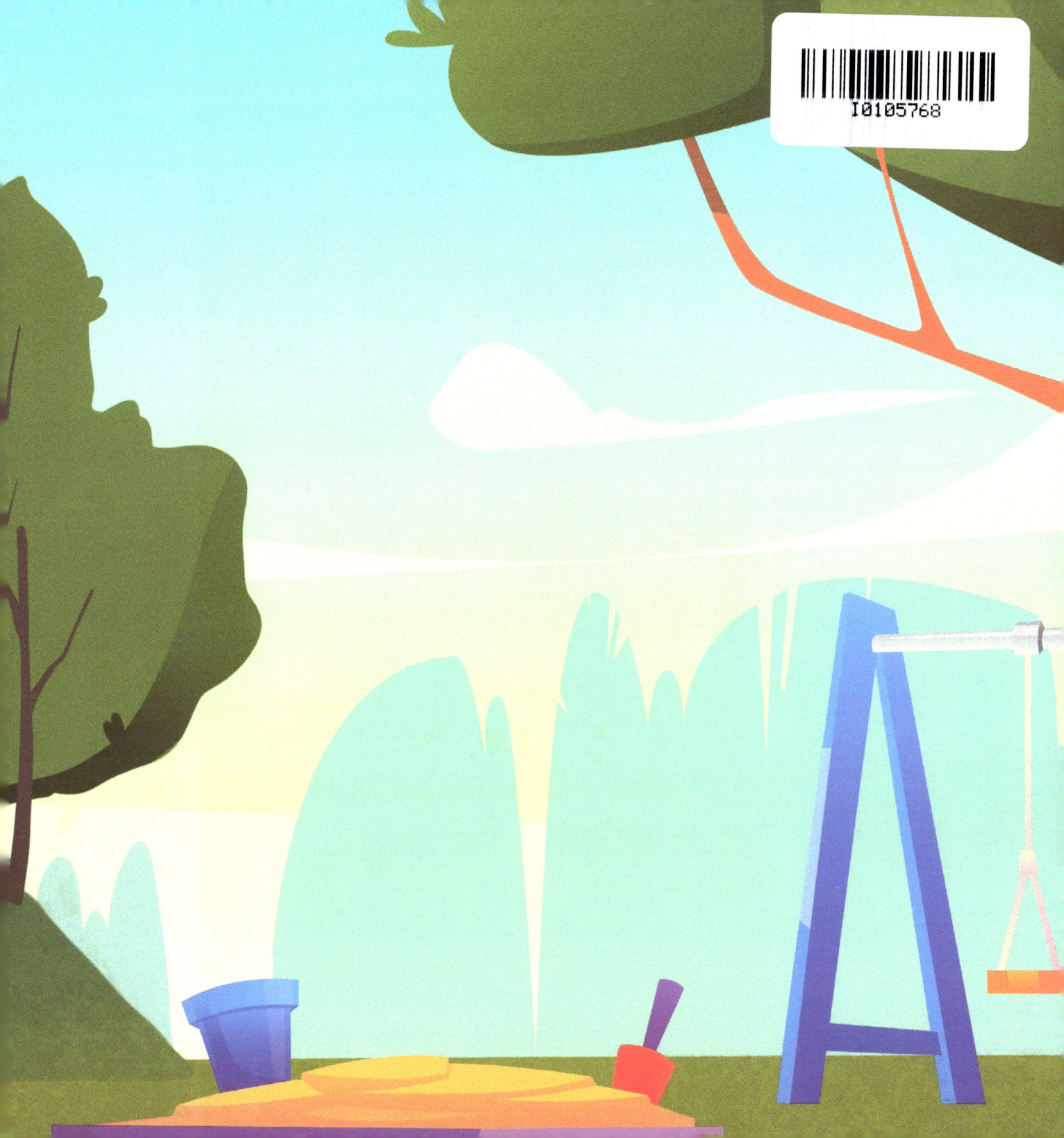

To my wonderful children and husband.
You all are my inspiration!

And to my amazing illustrator: Kseniya Bratukhina. You brought my story to life!

Cherrie

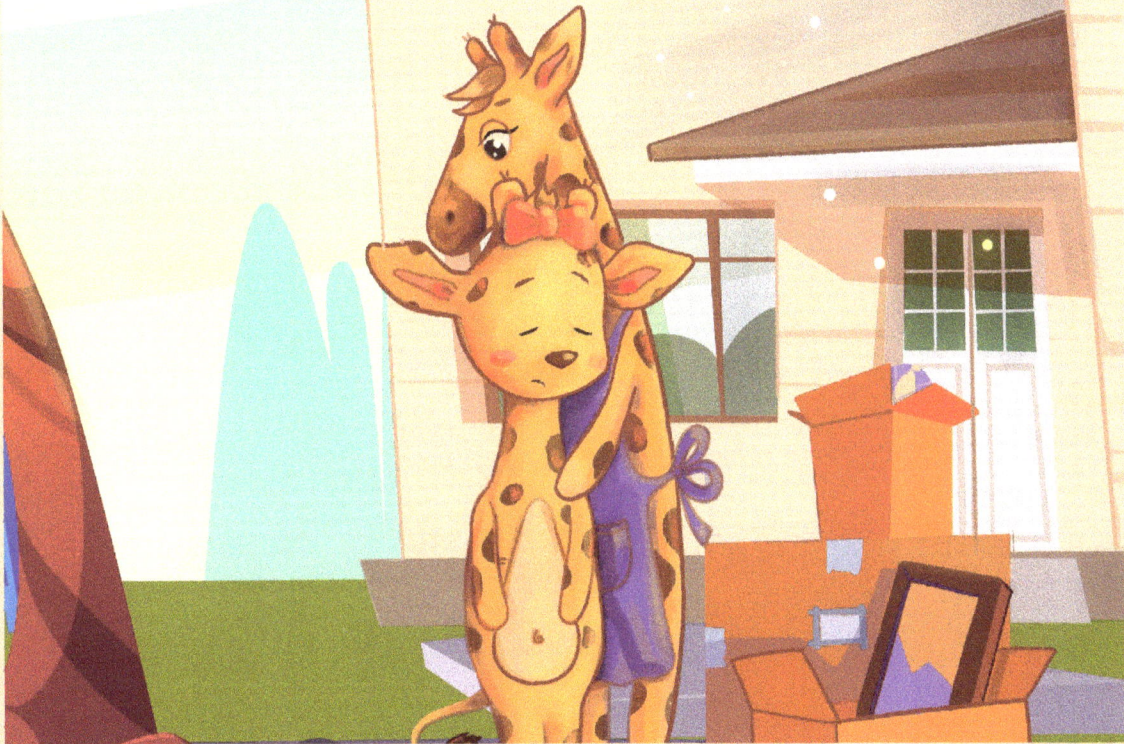

Cherrie Masai was sad.
She was moving away from all of
her friends to a new city where she
didn't know anyone.

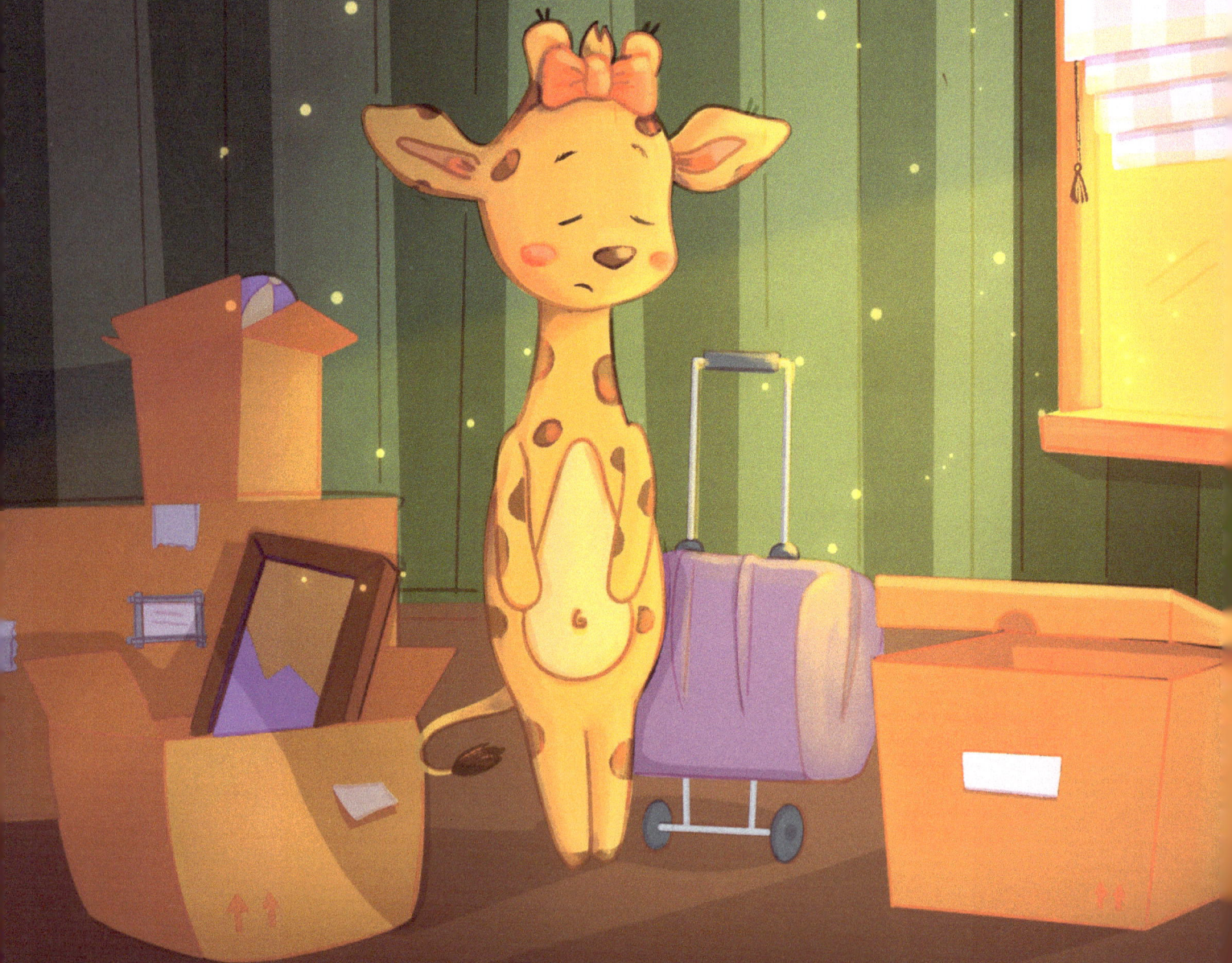

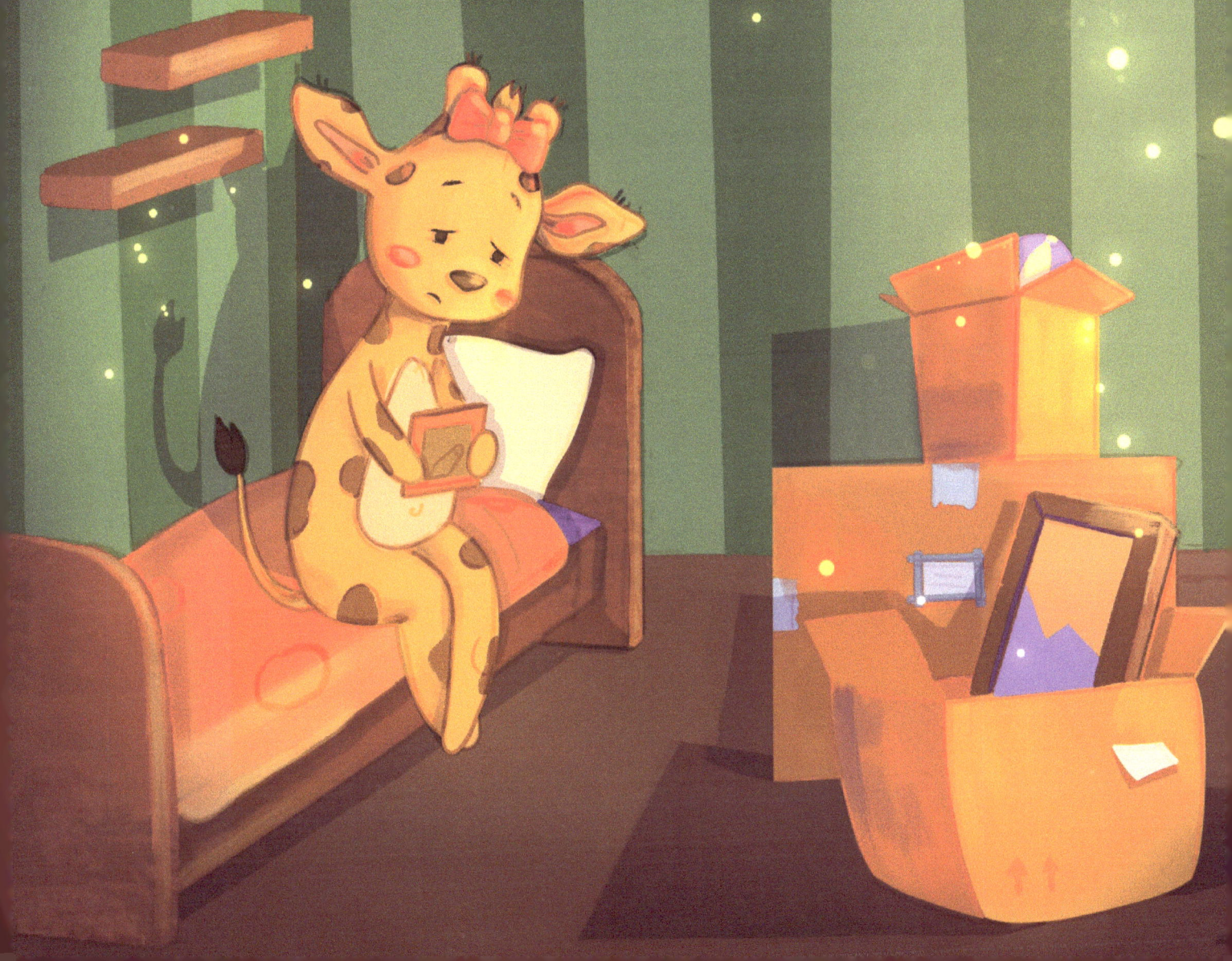

"Why do we have to move, mommy? All of my friends are here. And my favorite teacher is here. I don't want to go."

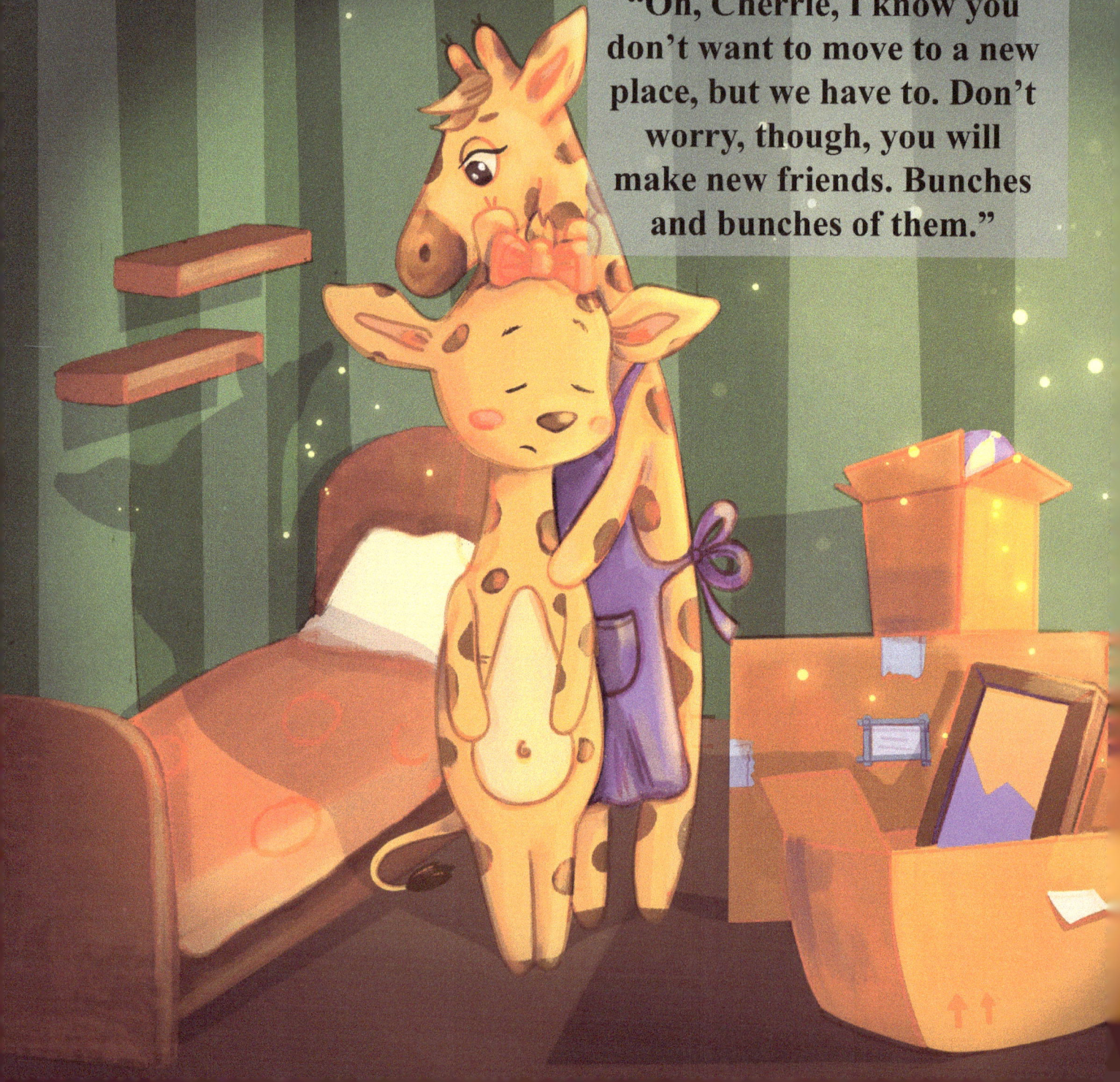

"Oh, Cherrie, I know you don't want to move to a new place, but we have to. Don't worry, though, you will make new friends. Bunches and bunches of them."

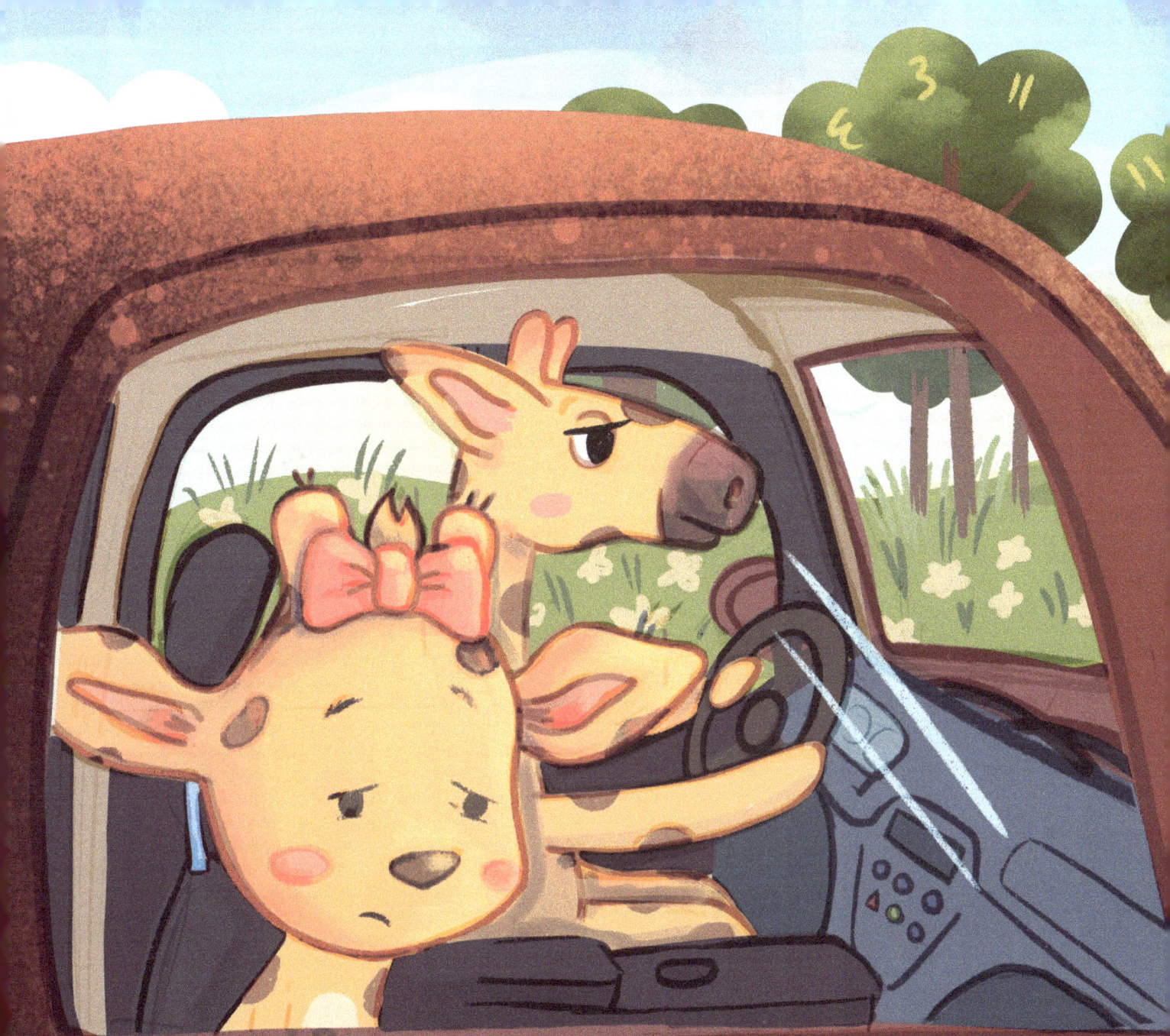

But her mommy's words didn't help. She was still sad as she drove away from her old house, her favorite park, and her friends.

"Look how big your new room is! And it's your favorite color! Oh, and look at this, you can see all the way to the park from your window! How about you go check it out after you get done unpacking?"

Cherrie looked down to the floor where she was opening up another box. She didn't want to go to the new park. She wouldn't know anyone there. She just knew that she wouldn't have any fun.

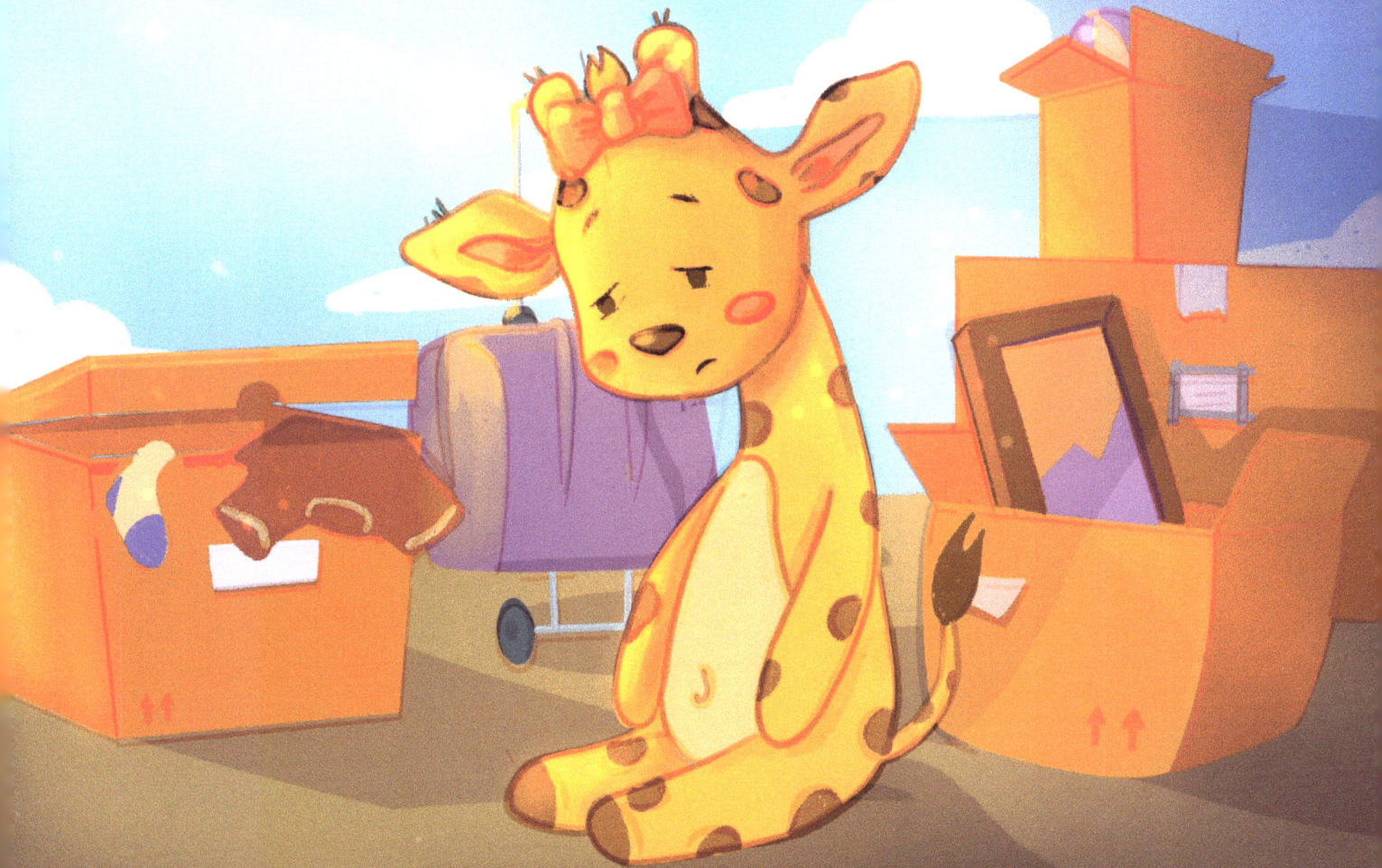

"Cherrie, why didn't you go to the park today? It was so sunny and warm outside," her mommy asked that night at dinner.

"I don't have any friends here, so I wouldn't have anyone to play with. I don't want to go all by myself," Cherrie complained.

Cherrie's mommy held up her hand and said, "Hold that thought." Then she walked into her bedroom.

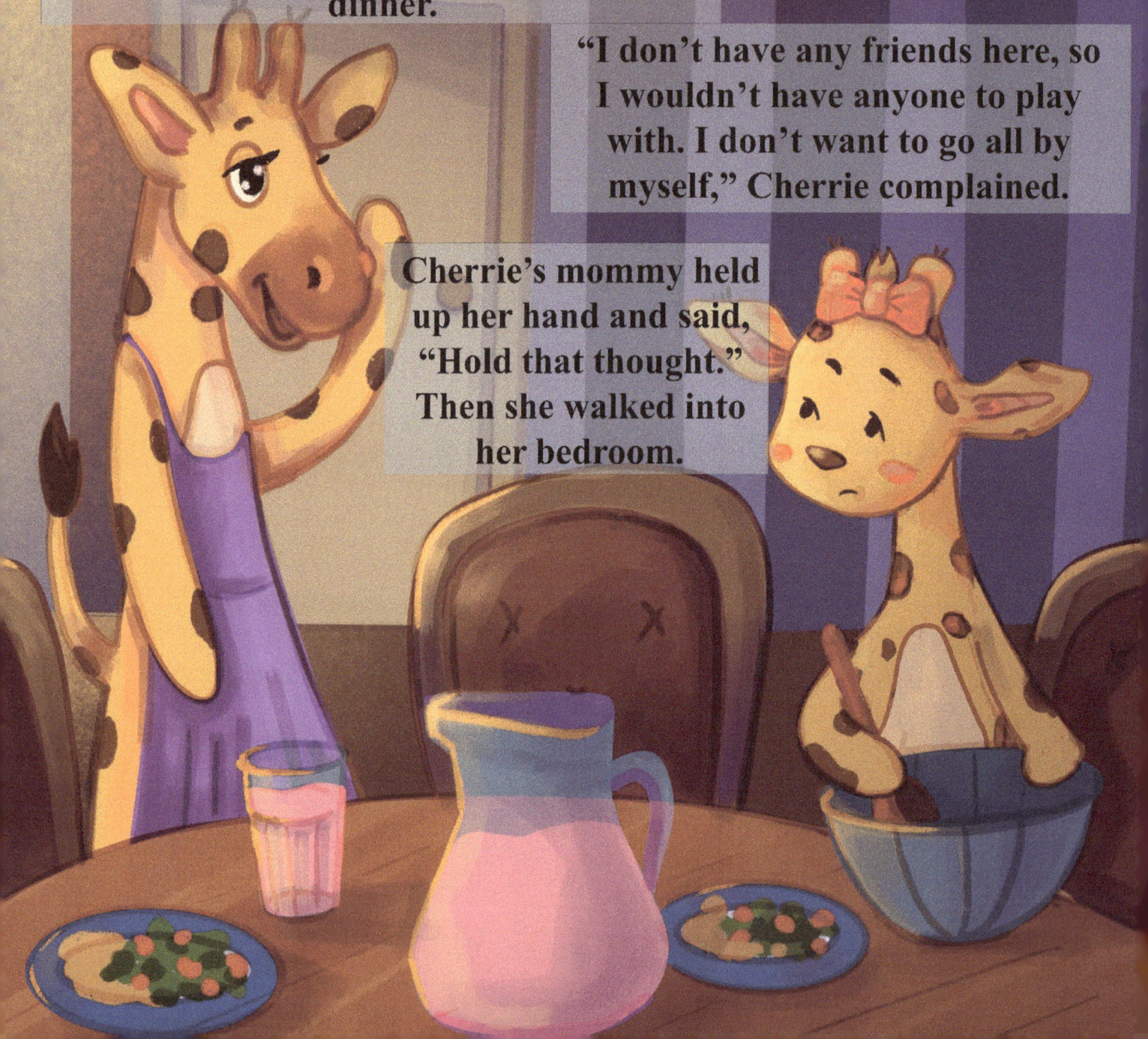

When she walked back in, she was holding a little, yellow stuffed bird. "Here," she said, handing it to Cherrie. "Now you will have a friend to play with at the park."

Cherrie looked at it but didn't take it. "Mommy, that's just a toy."

"Oh no, she is much more than just a toy. She was my best friend. When I was a child, she and I went on many, many great adventures!
And now you can too, if you just believe."

The next day, Cherrie took her new toy to the park.

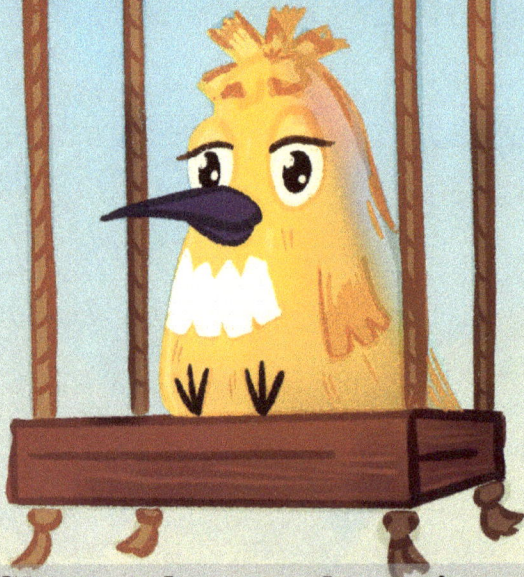

She put her on the swing, but she wouldn't swing.

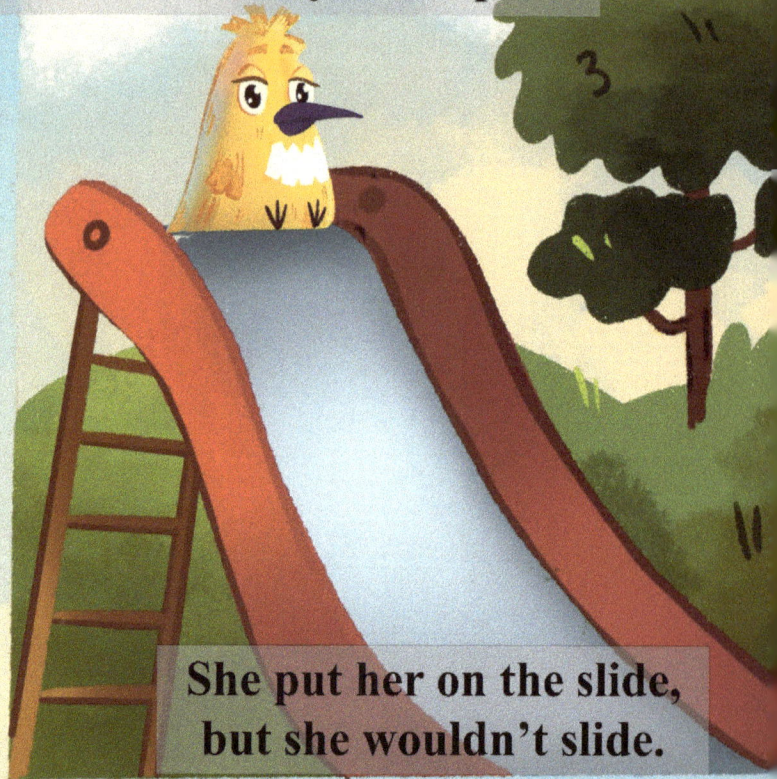

She put her on the slide, but she wouldn't slide.

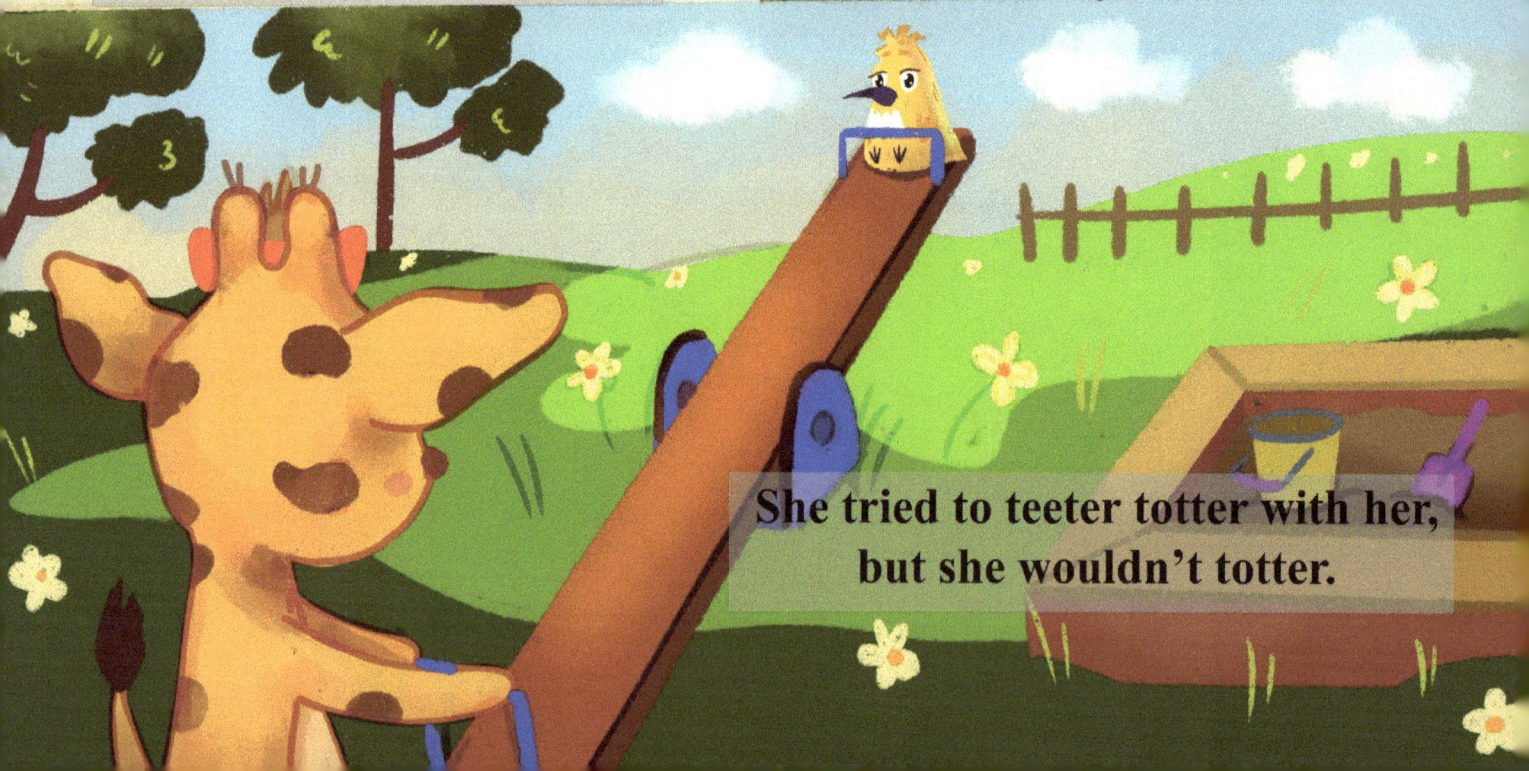

She tried to teeter totter with her, but she wouldn't totter.

Cherrie got mad because her new friend wasn't playing with her. Tired of playing at the park all by herself, Cherrie decided to go exploring in the woods instead.
She was kicking a pebble and hadn't gone too far down the path when she saw a small well.

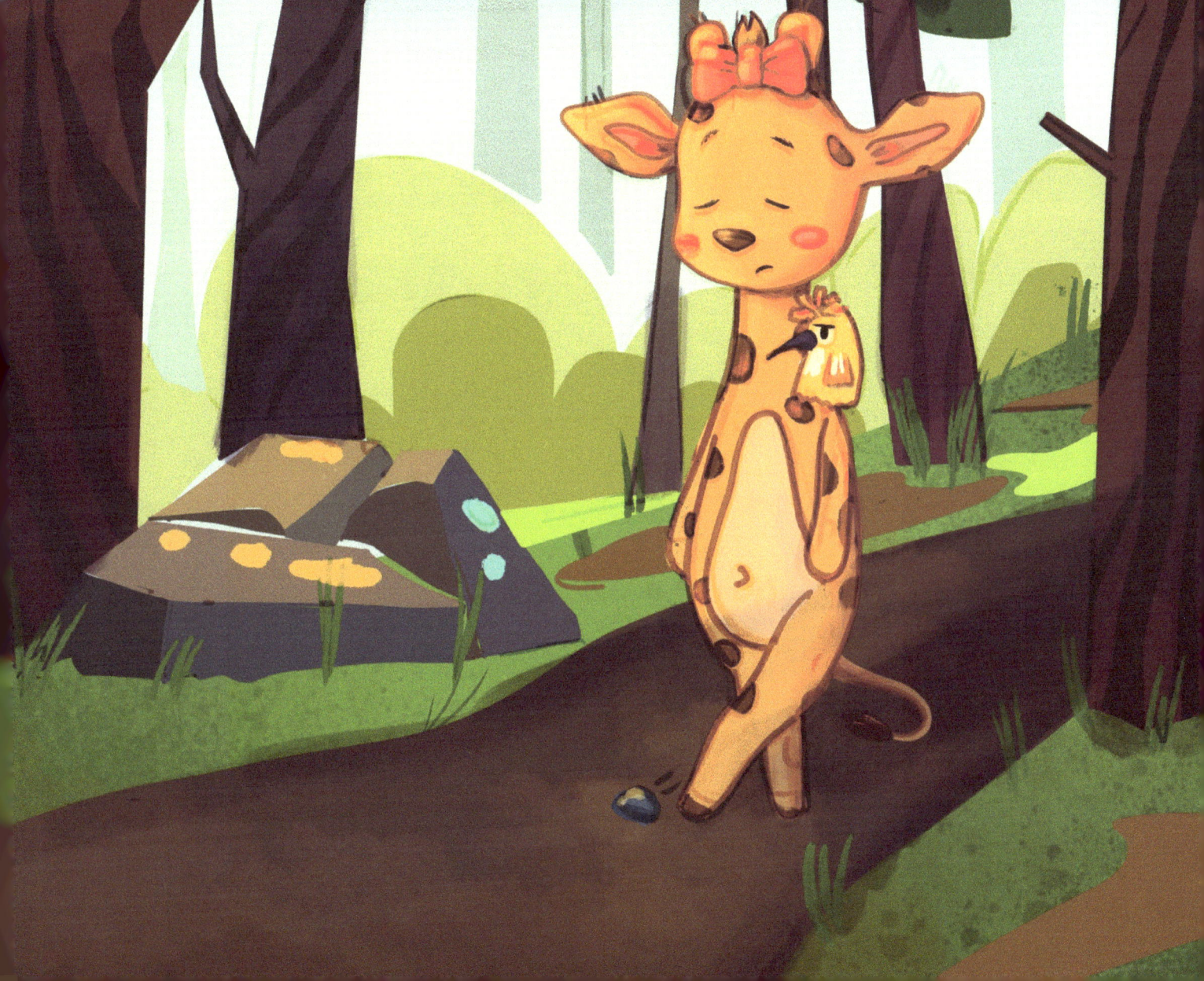

To grant the wish of desires within
Take a penny and drop it in.
Open your mind and close your eyes
And search the wants you hold inside.
If you believe and do not doubt
You will drop a penny in, and your wish
will come out.

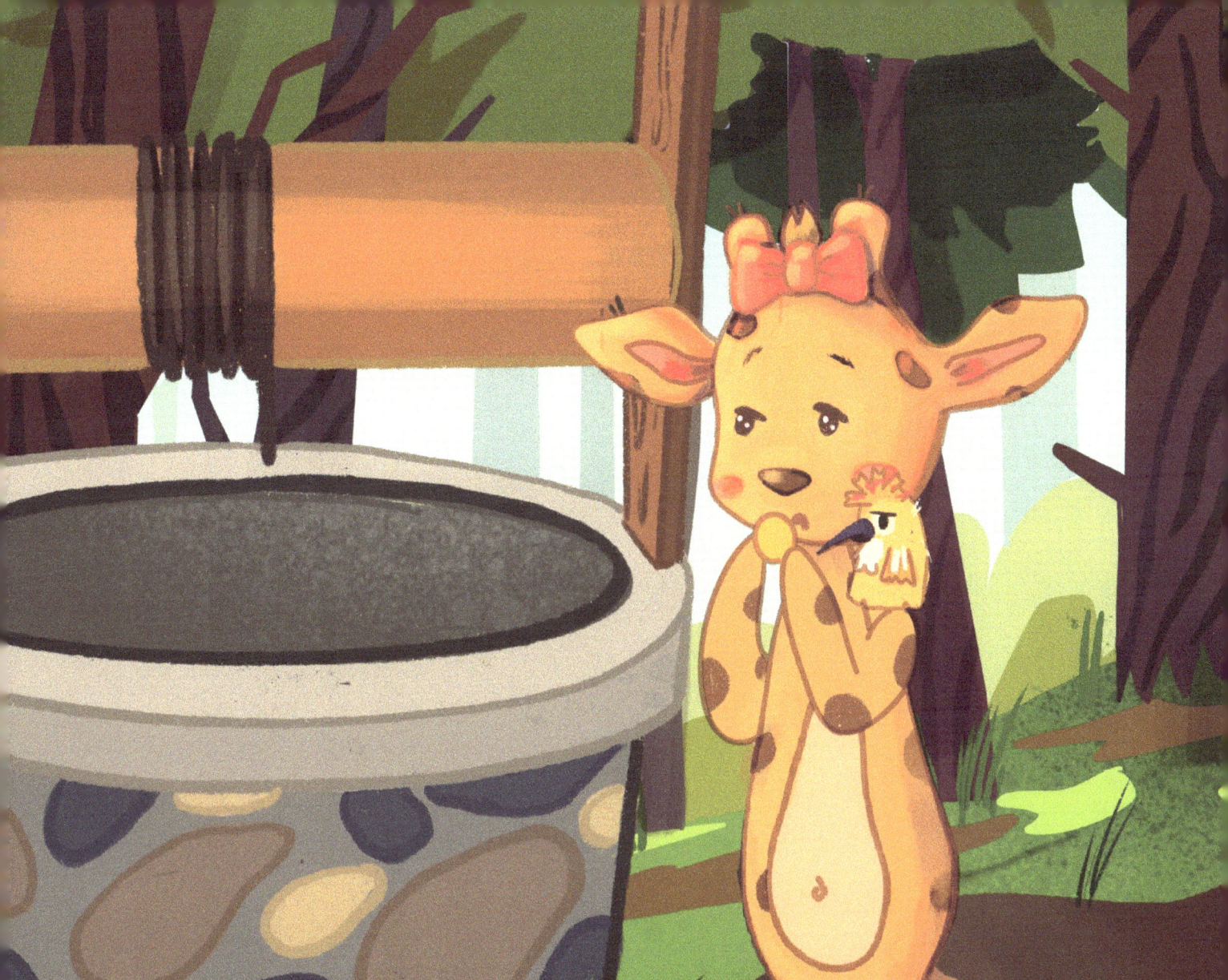

Cherrie didn't have a penny. So she rushed home, asked her
mom for one, and ran back as fast as she could. She held her
penny up to her mouth and whispered her wish.
"I wish I had a friend." She looked at the stuffed animal.
"I wish I had a real friend." She kissed her penny and
dropped it into the well.

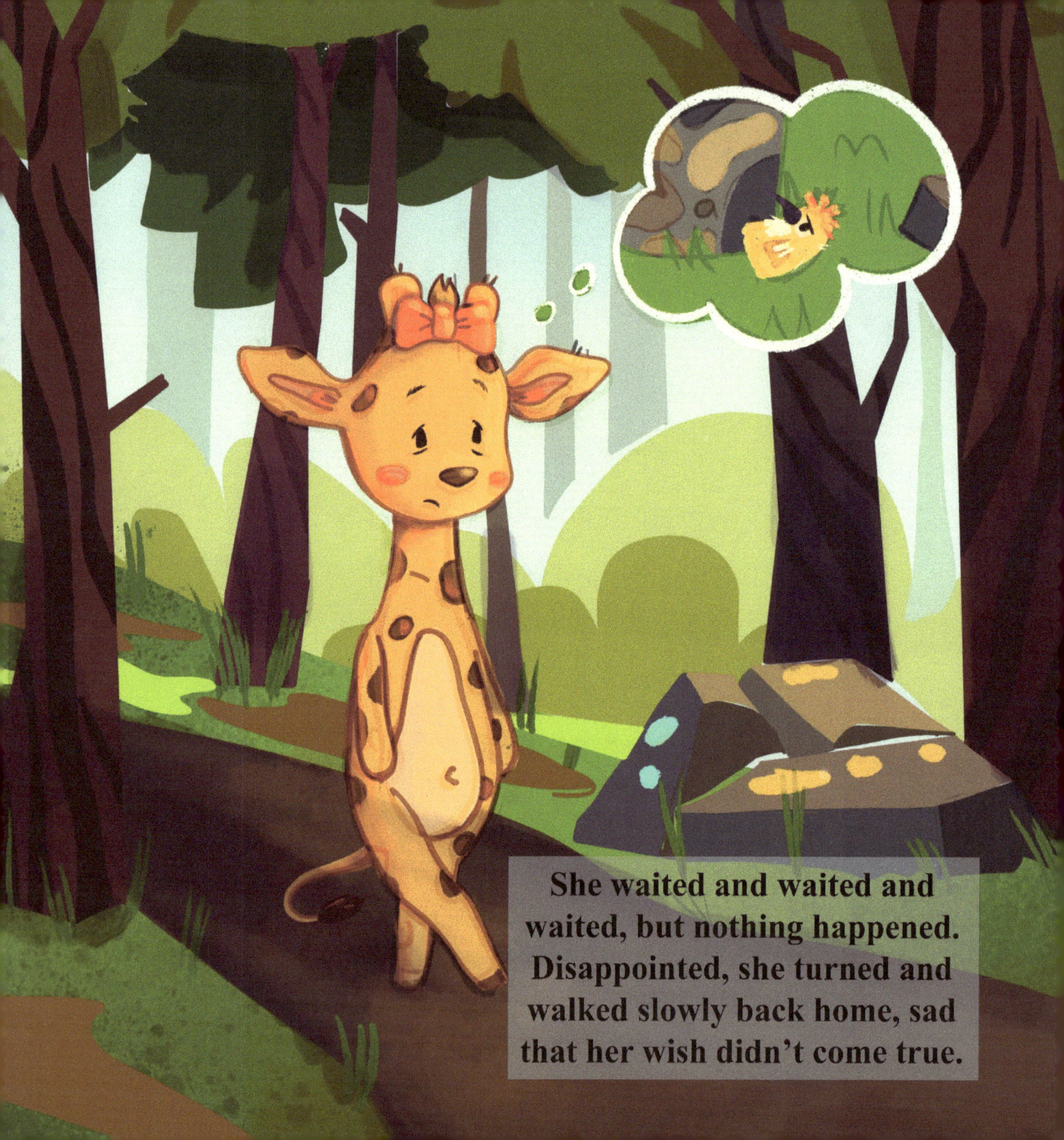

She waited and waited and waited, but nothing happened. Disappointed, she turned and walked slowly back home, sad that her wish didn't come true.

The next morning, Cherrie thought about going back to the park to play but pulled the covers over her head instead. She was still upset that she didn't get the friend she wished for.

"Time for breakfast," her mommy called.

Cherrie sighed, went to eat breakfast, then lay back down in her bed. Her mommy had asked if she was going to the park again, but she said no. She didn't want to go outside when she didn't have anyone to play with. She didn't want to do anything but sleep.

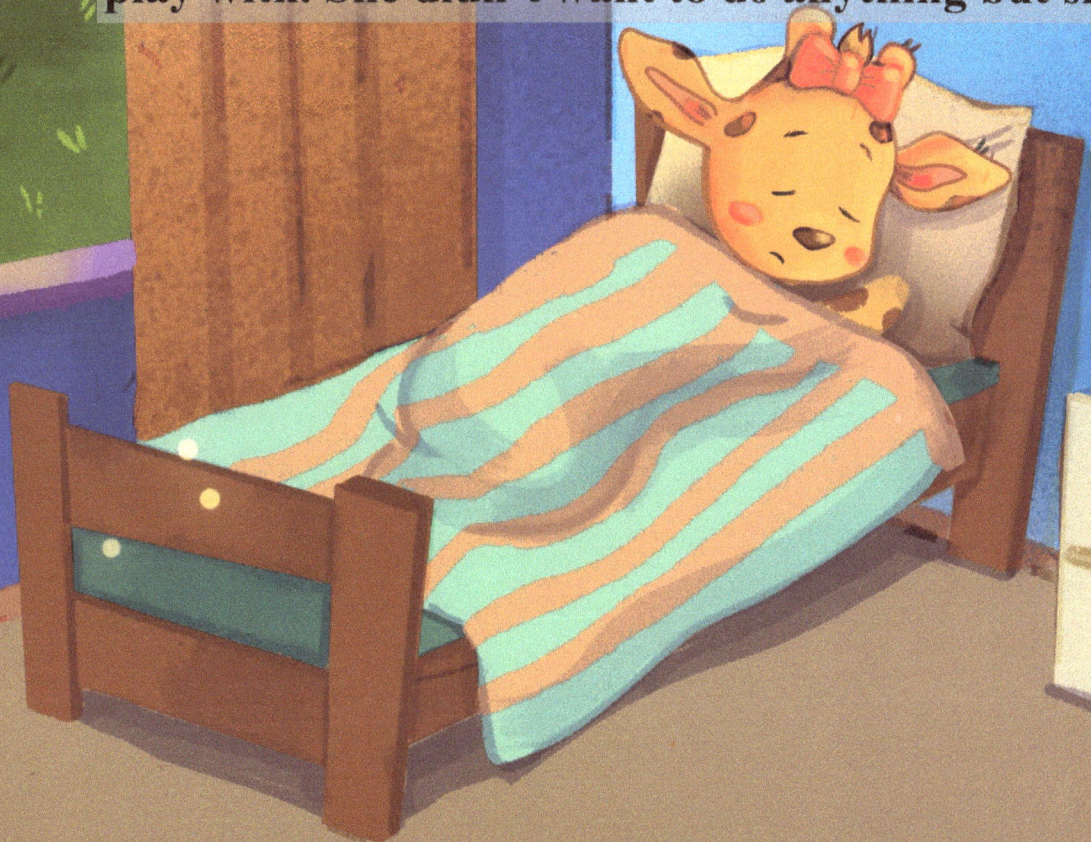

"Get up, sleepy head!"
"Who said that?" Cherrie asked, sitting up in bed.
"I did."
"Who?"
"Me!" the voice said, giggling.

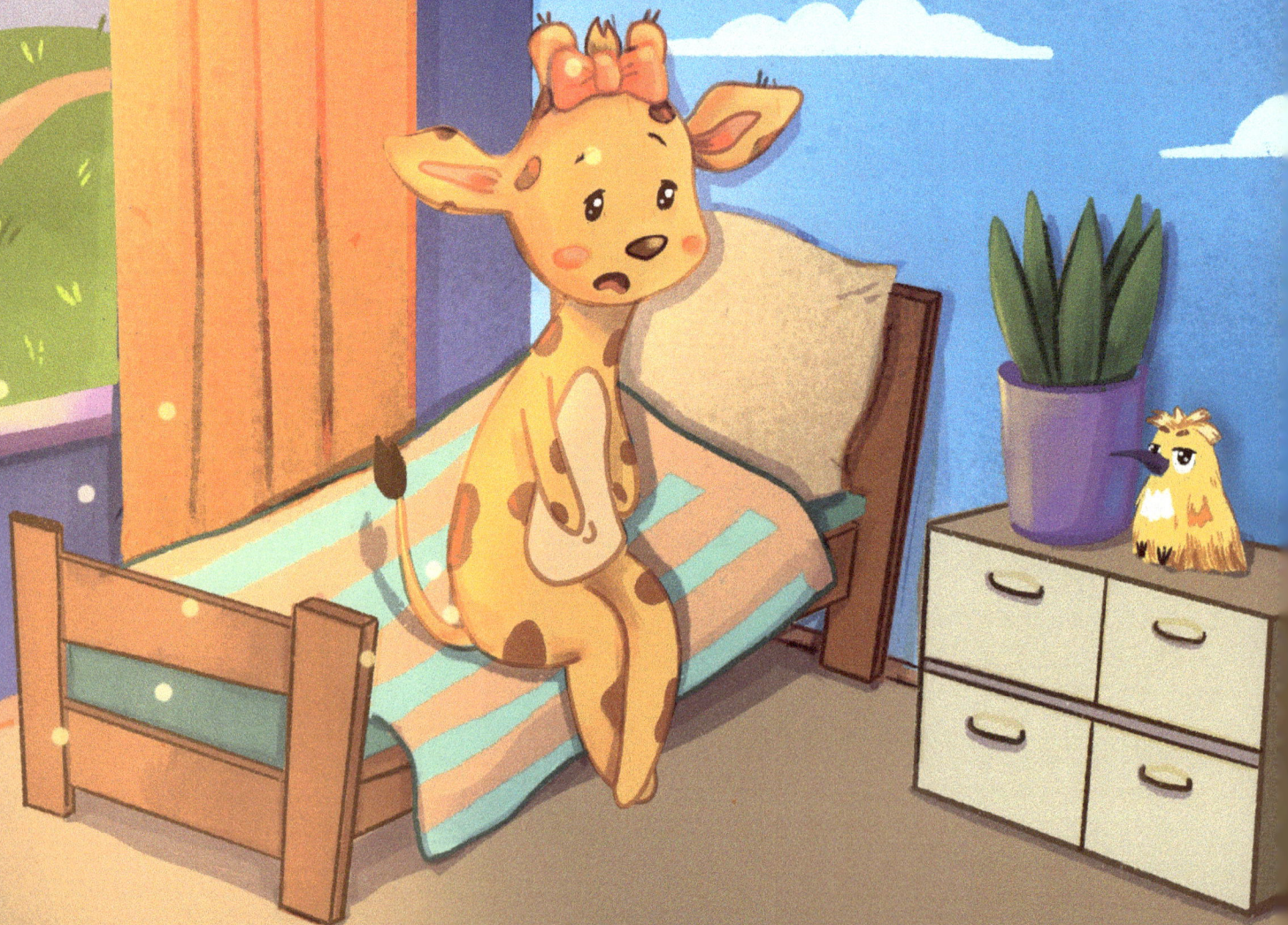

"Who is, 'Me'?" Cherrie asked, peering at the little bird.
She jumped and fell backwards when it flew up in the air and said, "I'm me! You wished for a friend, so here I am! Now we can do all kinds of fun stuff together!"

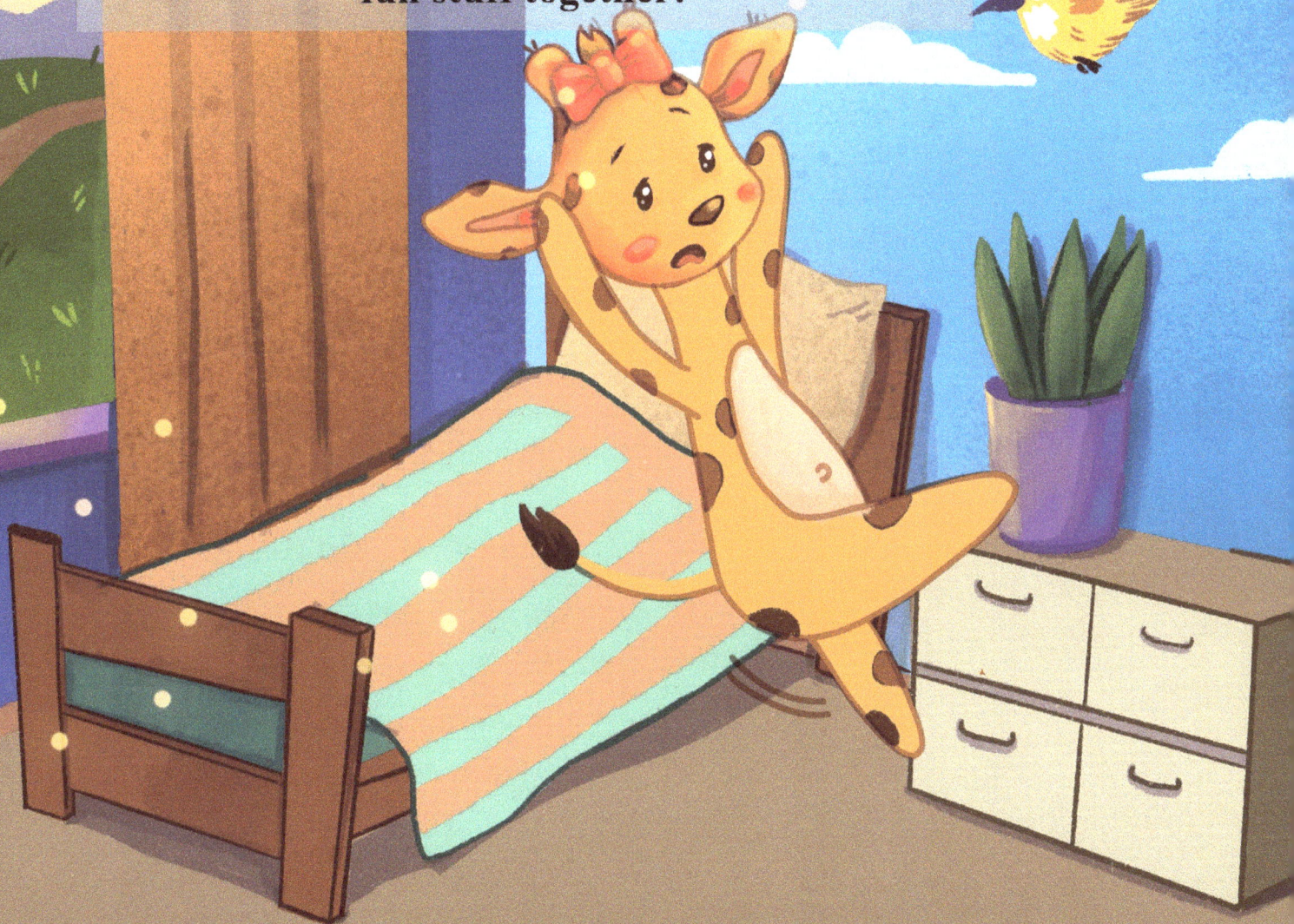

Cherrie was a little afraid, but happy at the same time. She had wanted a friend to play with, now she had one!

"What's your name?" she asked.
"My name is Harmony," the little bird answered.
"Mine is Cherrie."
"I already know that, silly," she laughed.

Cherrie was confused. "How do you already know my name?"

Harmony flew down and landed on her nose.

"We met when your mommy first gave you to me."

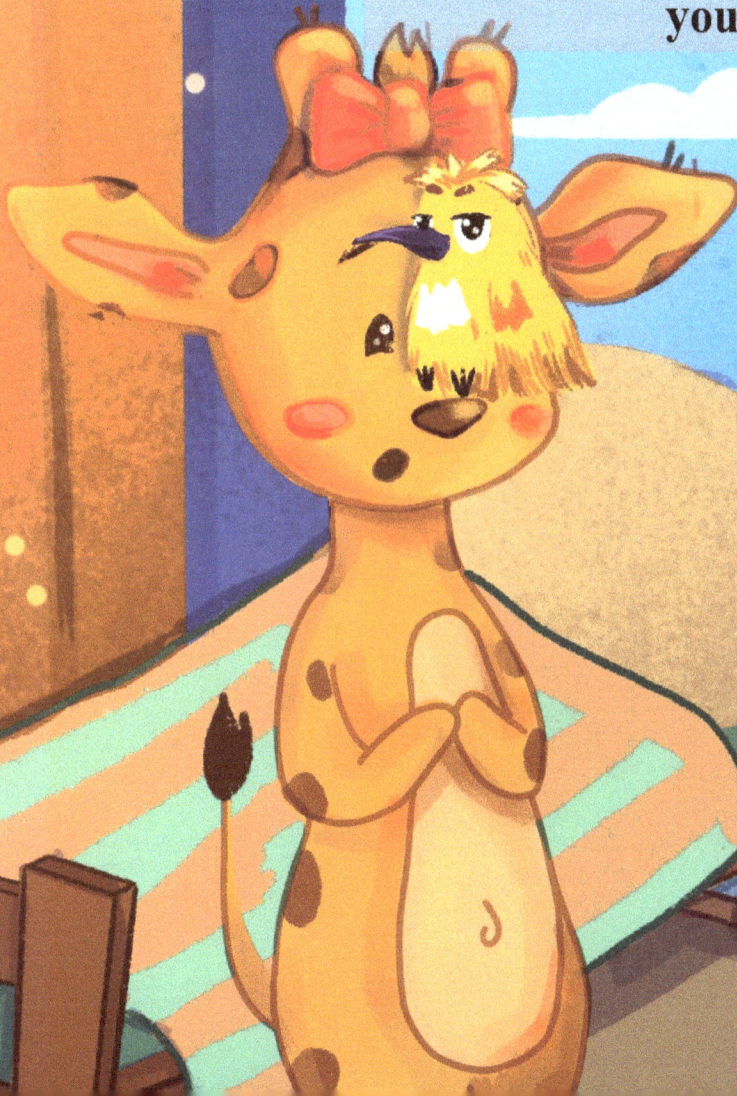

"But, how come you can talk and play with me now, but you didn't when I took you to the park," Cherrie asked.

"I couldn't until you made the wish. As I was laying on the ground by the well and watching you walk away from me, I got really sad. I was sad because you were sad. I wanted to holler after you, but I couldn't. And then after I couldn't see you anymore, a got really, really scared, especially when a really big dog came by and thought I was a toy for him to play with."

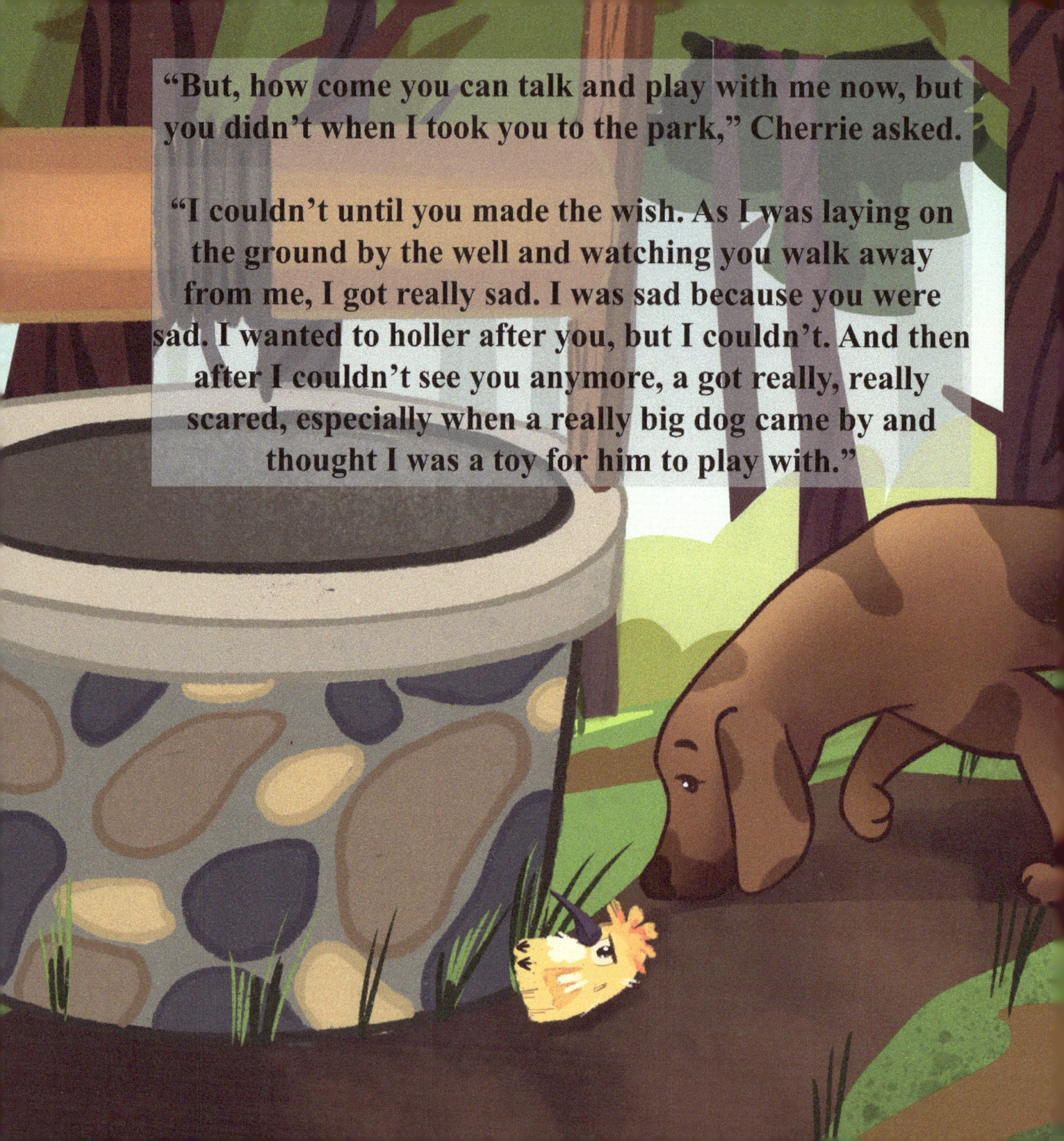

"Right as he was about to bite into me, all of a sudden I could move! I flew up so fast the he jumped back and started barking at me! I had to wait in a tree for a super long time until he decided to leave. Then I came looking for you. My best friend."

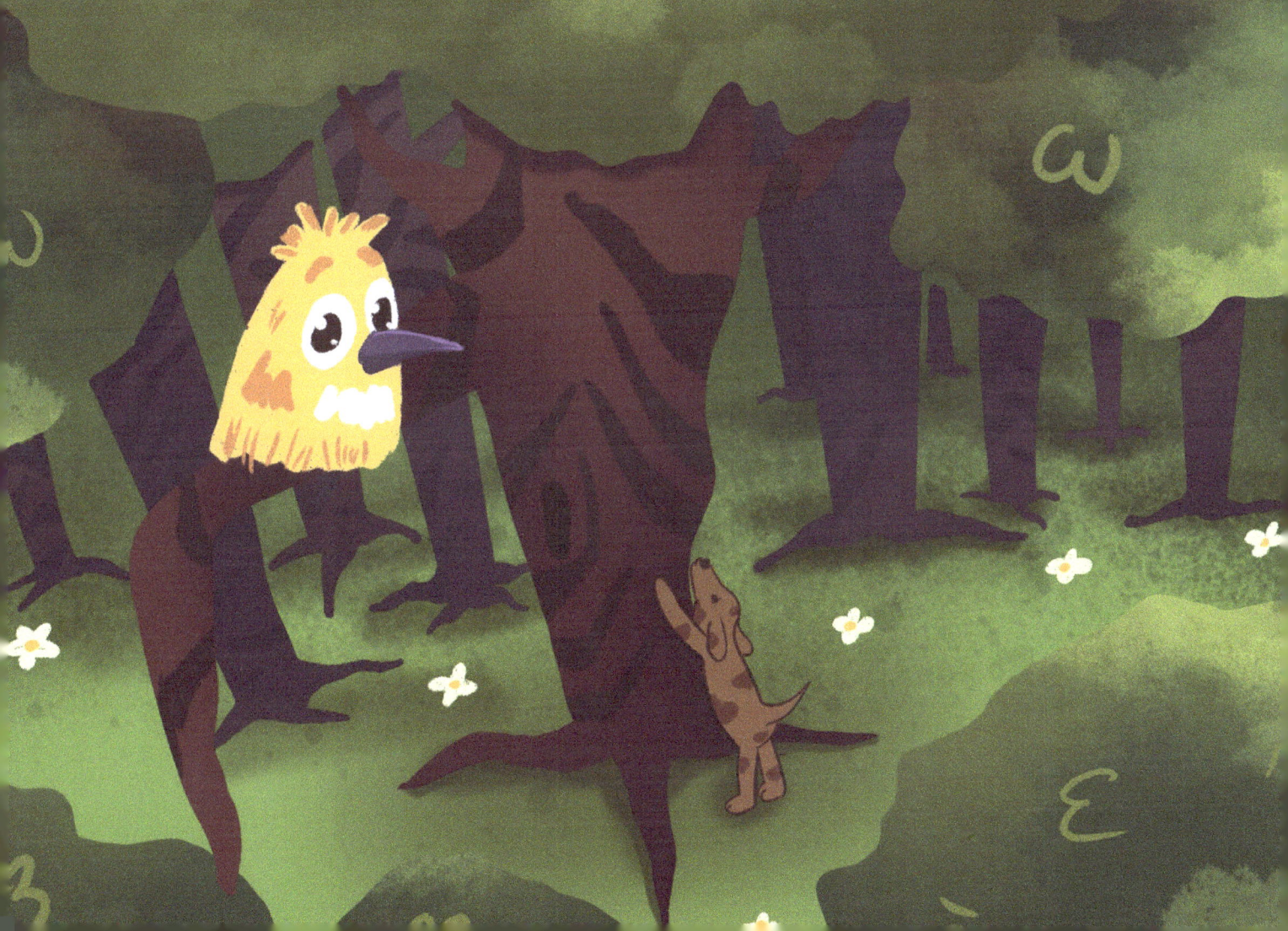

"I'm sorry I left you there," Cherrie said. "I didn't know you were real. I just thought you were a toy that my mommy gave me. I wanted a friend so much and when you couldn't play with me, I got upset. I used to have friends, but then I moved here and don't have any anymore."

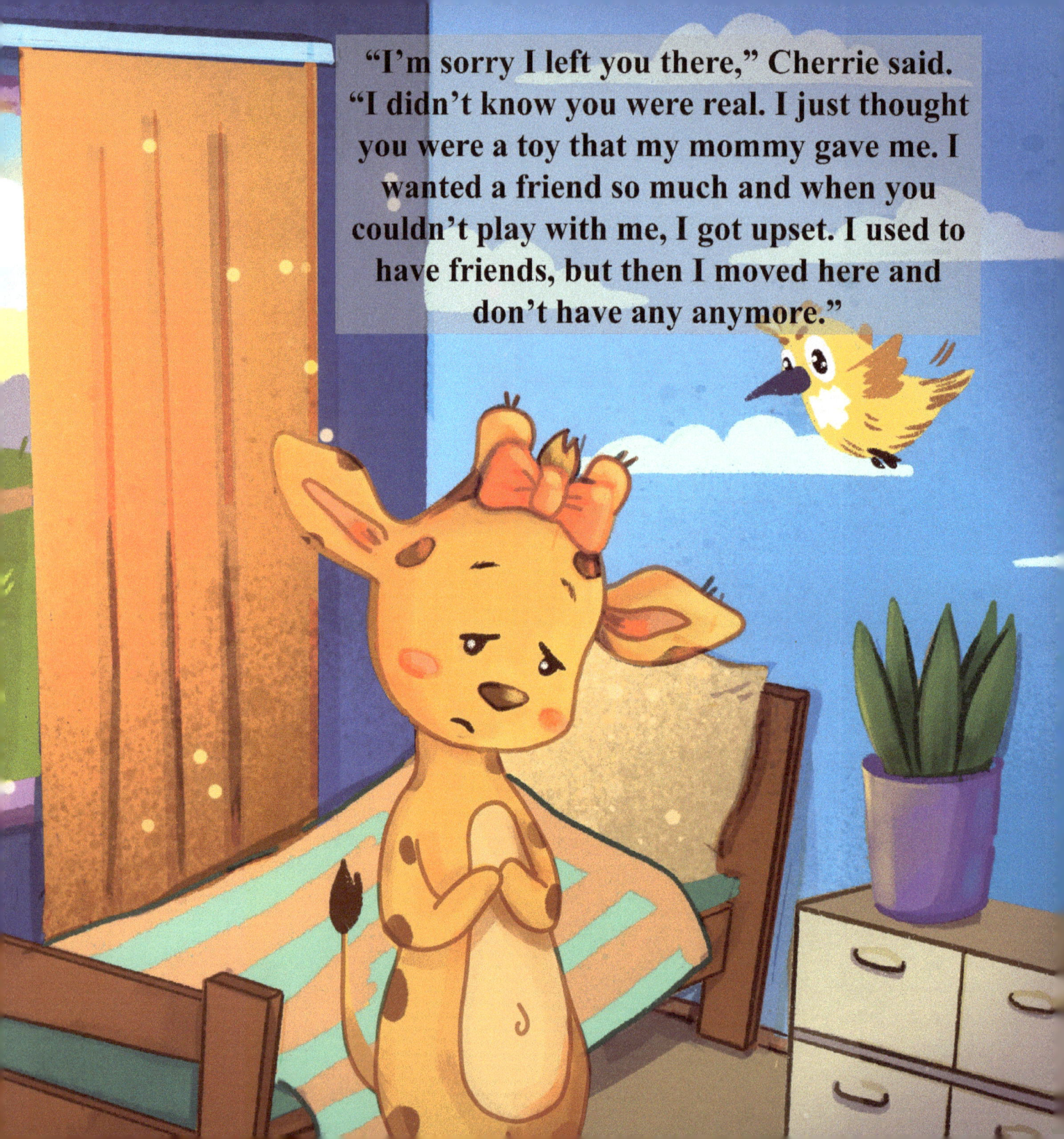

"Don't be sad! I know you didn't know I was real. But now you do! And now you have a friend! Now we can have so much fun! We can go on adventures and do all sorts of new things!"

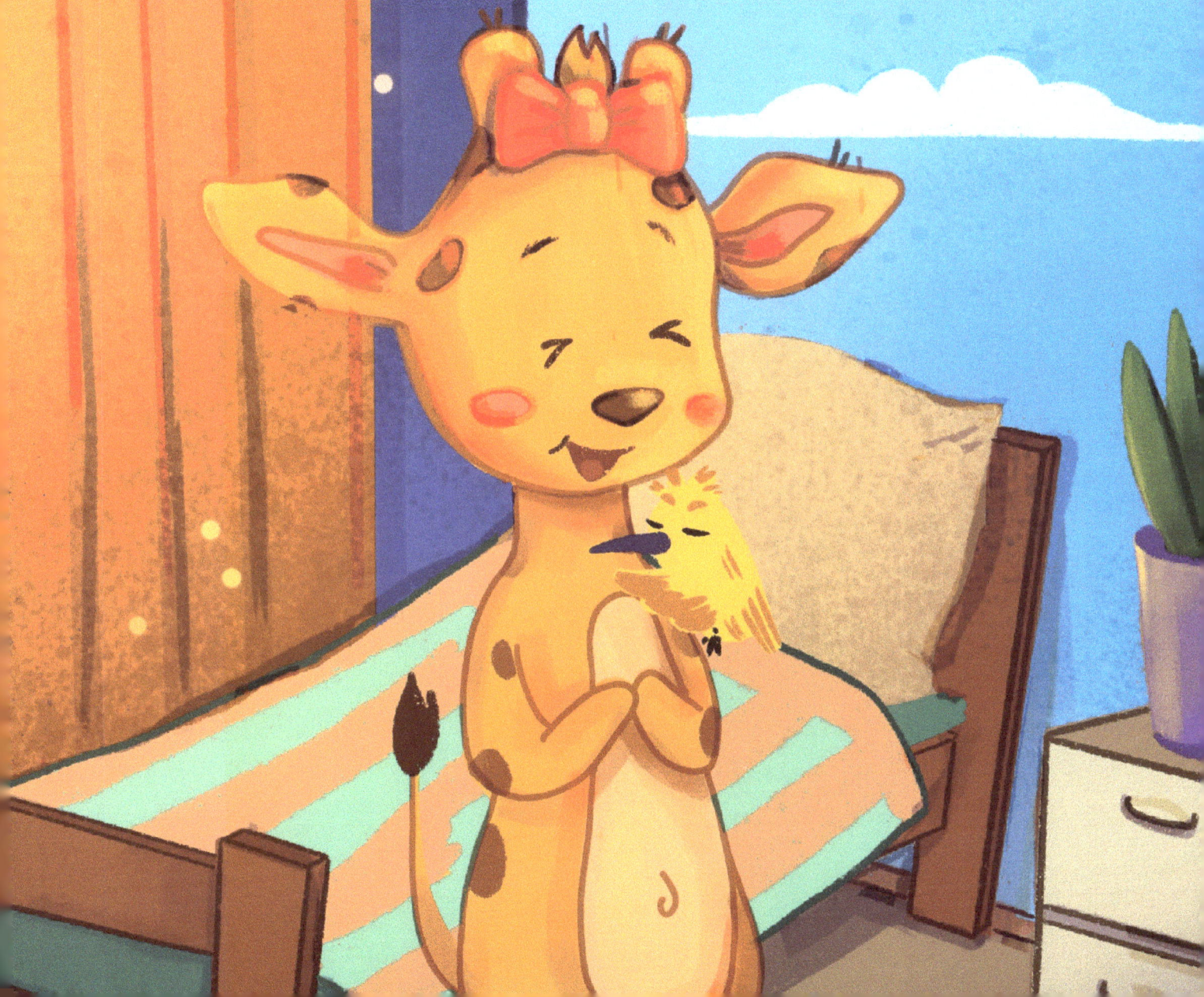

Cherrie got ready as quickly as she could before rushing downstairs to give her mommy a big hug. "Thank you for giving me Harmony, mommy. I love her so much! We are going to go to the park to have an adventure now, OK?"

Her mommy hugged her back and asked, "Who is Harmony?"
"The stuffed toy you gave me yesterday. See?" Cherrie pointed to the spot where Harmony was flying.
"Oh, yeah, of course. Nice to meet you, Harmony." She waved to a spot on the other side of where Harmony was. You two go and have fun!"

"Why didn't she see you?" Cherrie asked as they walked to the park.
"Only kids can see me move and talk," Harmony said.
"But why?"
"I don't really know why. It's just always been like that. Now come on, let's go have an adventure!"

Cherrie didn't ask any more questions. She played on the swings. She played on the slides. She had many great adventures with her new best friend.

One night while she was lying in bed, she heard a loud bang outside. Cherrie jumped and ran to the living room where her mommy was.

"What was that loud bang?" she asked.

"That's our new neighbors moving in next door," her mommy said.

Cherrie rushed to the window and looked outside. What she saw made her smile.

"I can't wait until tomorrow," Cherrie told Harmony when they got back to her room. Harmony swirled in a happy circle. "Me, too!"

"I'll see if he wants to come to the park with us tomorrow. Then he can go on our adventures with us," Cherrie said, laying back down on her bed. "Tomorrow we will get another friend."

"And friendship is such a grand adventure," Harmony said, snuggling down on the pillow next to her.

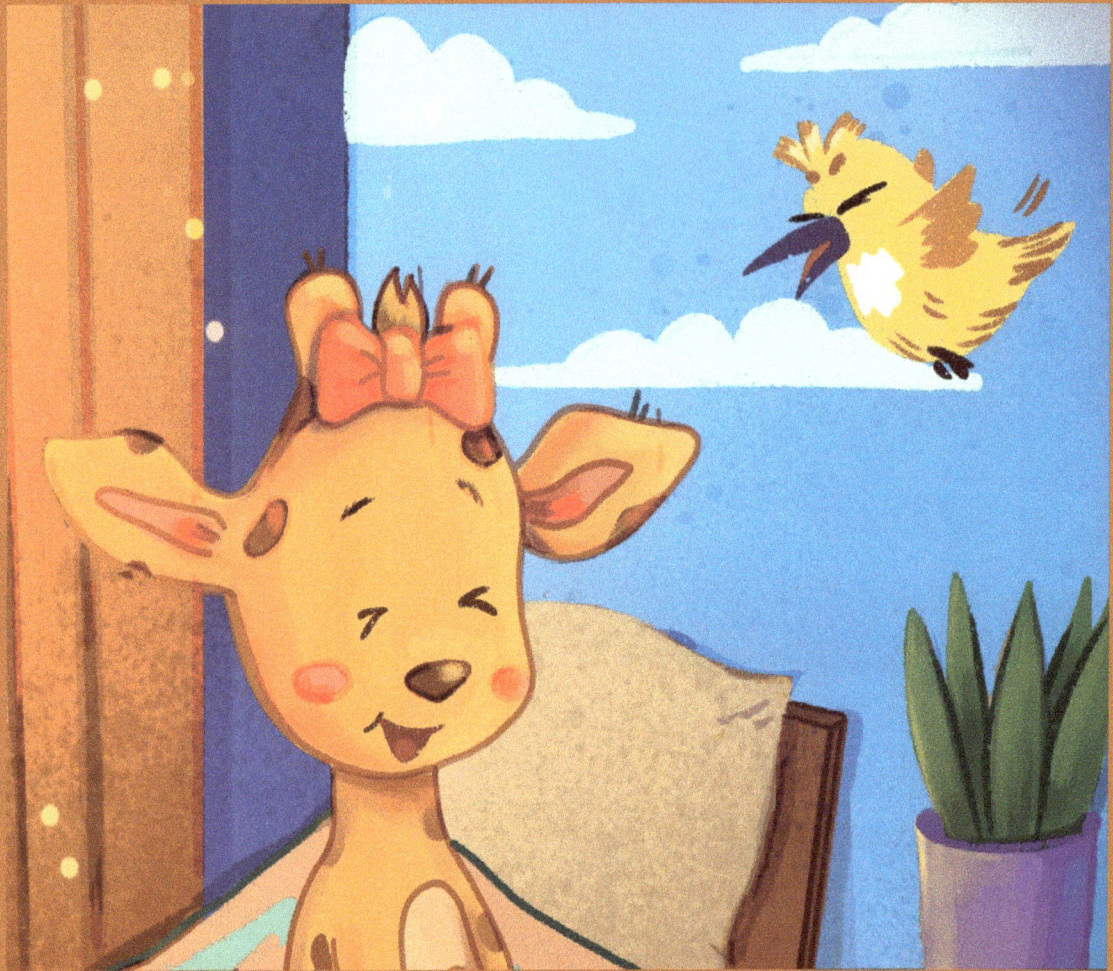

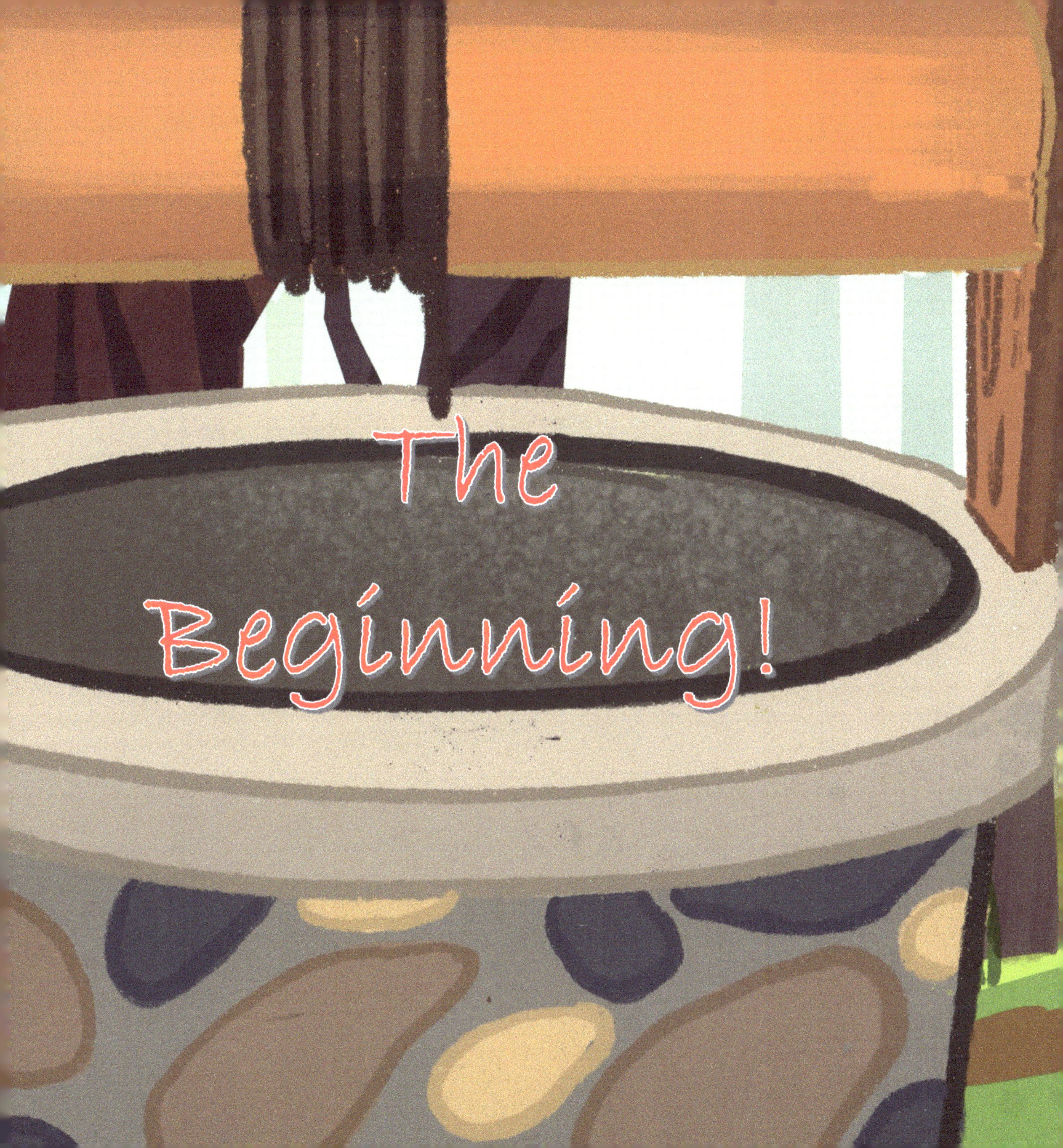

The
Beginning!

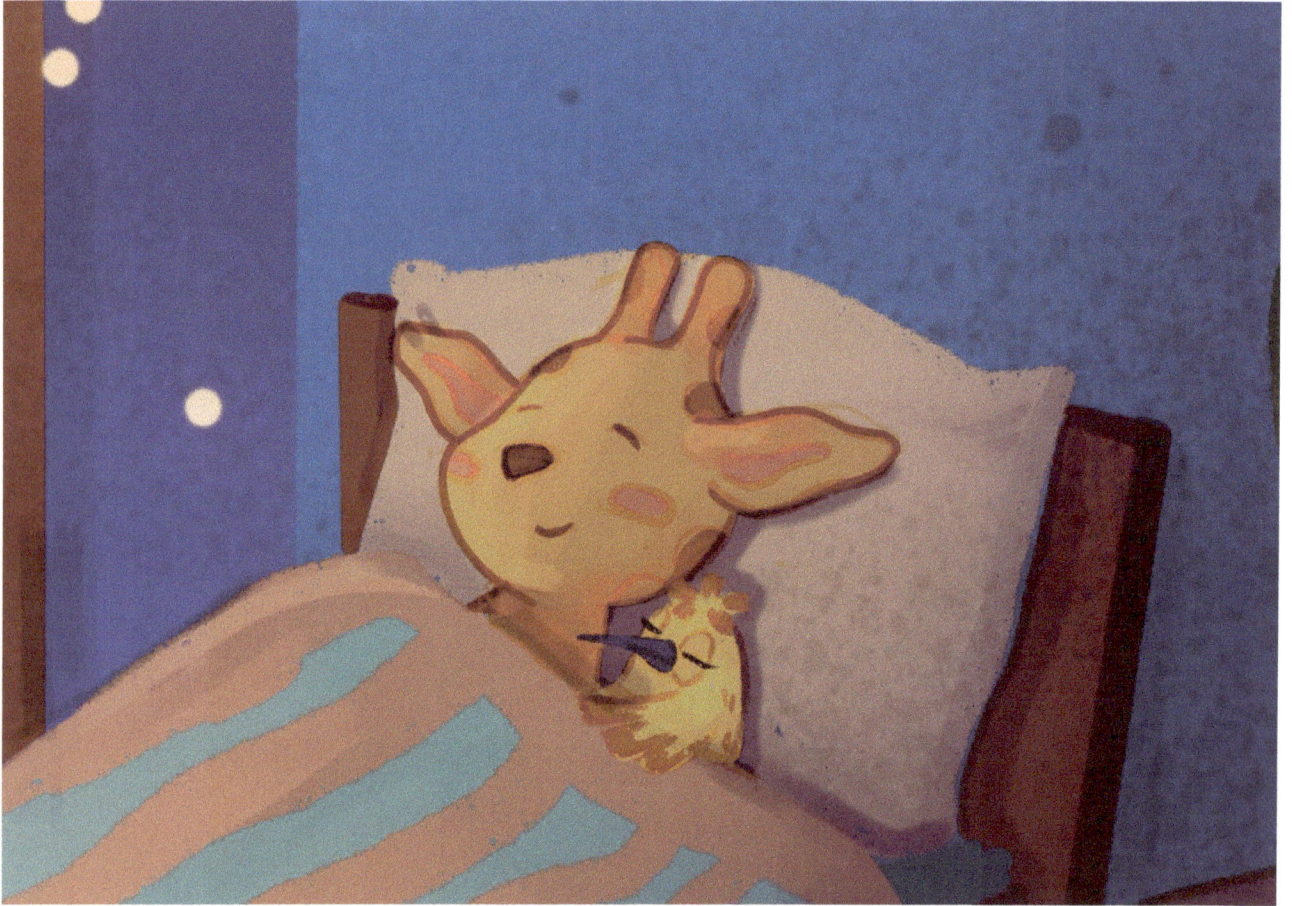

Many thanks to my wonderful illustrator:

Kseniya Bratukhina.

If you would like to utilize her amazing talent, you can contact her at:

kbratukhina@stayaproduction.com

www.ingramcontent.com/pod-product-compliance
Lightning Source LLC
Chambersburg PA
CBHW042344030426
42335CB00030B/3450